Borderline Personality Disorder

The Ultimate Borderline Personality Disorder Survival Guide

How To Live With Someone With BPD With Your Sanity Intact

Sylvia Jacob

Your Free Gift

As a way of thanking you for the purchase, I'd like to offer you a complimentary gift:

- **5 Pillar Life Transformation Checklist:** This short book is about life transformation, presented in bit size pieces for easy implementation. I believe that without such a checklist, you are likely to have a hard time implementing anything in this book and any other thing you set out to do religiously and sticking to it for the long haul. It doesn't matter whether your goals relate to weight loss, relationships, personal finance, investing, personal development, improving communication in your family, your overall health, finances, improving your sex life, resolving issues in your relationship, fighting PMS successfully, investing, running a successful business, traveling etc. With a checklist like this one, you can bet that anything you do will seem a lot easier to implement until the end. Therefore, even if you don't continue reading this book, at least read the one thing that will help you in every other aspect of your life. Grab your copy now by clicking/tapping here or simply enter http://bit.ly/2fantonfreebie into your browser. Your life will never be the same again (if you implement what's in this book), I promise.

PS: I'd like your feedback. If you are happy with this book, please leave a review on Amazon.

Introduction

Borderline Personality Disorder is a mental health condition that makes it difficult for a person to control their emotions and reactions to day-to-day life events and challenges.

Everyone has a portion of their brain, the Amygdala that controls the fight-or-flight response. When there is a looming threat, this part of your brain sends distress signals to your sympathetic nervous system, and helps you decide how to respond to the challenge.

But for a person suffering from Borderline Personality Disorder, it's almost like their fight-or-flight switch can be tripped on by everything and anything, even by things that would not be considered a threat by other.

Everything feels more scary and stressful for them than it does for regular people and because they also have mood disorders and challenges with their thought process and image, they can be very difficult people to live, work or fall in love with.

The good news is that Borderline Personality is a treatable condition. There are a lot of effective treatments and therapies that can alleviate the symptoms of this disorder so your loved one doesn't have to live with it forever.

However, before the treatments start working, you have to learn how to live with a person suffering from this disorder without losing yourself. You have to learn how to prevent and deal with conflicts, care for them, and set boundaries so that you don't lose your sanity while trying to help them get better.

In this book, you will learn:

✓ What Borderline Personality Disorder is

✓ How to tell that your loved one is indeed suffering from Borderline Personality Disorder

✓ How to Identify Triggers for Manic and Depressive Episodes and How to help them during mood episodes

✓ How to Manage and Reduce Conflicts in the relationships

✓ How to Care for Yourself and Set Boundaries

✓ Effective Treatments and Therapies for Borderline Personality Disorder

✓ And much, much more!

Let's begin!

Table of Contents

Chapter 1: It's Not Their Fault!

Saint and I have been married for 20 years.

I still get butterflies in my stomach when I remember how sweet our courtship was, especially the first few weeks following our meeting.

We first met at a friend's wedding. I was on the bridal train and he was a groomsman.

The night before the wedding, we organized a small party for the couple and Saint was chosen to pick us, the bridesmaids, from our hotel to the club where we were going to have the party.

On the way to the club, the other ladies made a joke about my hometown and everyone burst out laughing. I started to defend my town frantically and as he would tell me later, that was when he fell in love with me.

It was dark so I couldn't see his face but I could hear his voice clearly and I loved the way he sounded.

When we got to the club, I couldn't help but notice that he was more concerned about making sure that everyone else was comfortable, and got what they wanted. I think that was when I started to like him- I admired his sense of responsibility.

When it was time to dance, I wasn't interested and neither was he. We both sat across from each other in the VIP section, drinking and watching everyone dance.

Just as I was beginning to get bored of the party, he came up to me and asked that we dance. Since I already liked him, I didn't hesitate.

We got dancing and it was so romantic; it felt like we had known each other for years.

After the party, he dropped us off at the hotel and asked for my phone number. I refused to give it to him. I liked him but I didn't want a relationship at the time so I politely declined and walked away to nurse my hangover.

The next morning was the wedding and I was really busy with getting everything in order. I was like the auxiliary bridal planner, and a lot of responsibilities fell on my shoulders.

We had a nice wedding and just as I was settling in to enjoy the wedding reception, someone delivered unsettling news from the bride.

The bride was 'giving me the honor of delivering the toast'.

For me, that was no honor. I had a very terrible phobia for public speaking.

The thought of facing the guests to say anything with everyone staring at me and listening to what I had to say gave me the chills. I began to panic.

I tried to push the responsibility on other bridesmaids but none of them was keen on public speaking- they all rejected the honors.

Suddenly one of them said *"Why not ask Saint to do it for you?"*

"Uhhmm, who is Saint?" I asked, confused.

"The guy you were dancing with yesterday" she replied

"He'll do it?" I asked.

"Yeah, he was our student president in high school, he gives great speeches"

So off I went to find Saint and I didn't have to ask him twice. He laughed my Glossophobia off and suggested we give the toast together so I don't offend the bride.

We did it together and it was so beautiful, we got a standing ovation.

He asked for my phone number again but I still refused.

The bridesmaid who suggested I ask him to do the toast for me saw him trying to get my number and as soon as I sat down, she looked at me in a weird way, like she was concerned for me and said *"Saint? I hope you don't plan on dating Saint?"*

And before I had the chance to say anything else she quickly added *"Don't be fooled by his cuteness, that man is one crazy m*****f***er"*

"Crazy?" I asked, confused.

"Yeah, like sick in the head" She replied as she stood up to go dance.

She sounded like a disgruntled Ex to me so I didn't pay much attention to her. I thought, maybe they had some history and he hurt her feelings or something.

The third time Saint asked for my number, it would have been too ridiculous not to give it to him; I admired his persistence if nothing else.

We started a very hot and sweet romance and three weeks later, he invited me to visit him in his state, three hours from mine.

He had been nothing but sweet for three weeks and I had no qualms visiting him at all.

However, my first visit to him left me confused, and left a very sour taste in my mouth about the relationship.

Saint was very kind and sweet on the first day of my arrival. We kissed from the airport all the way home and we had a very romantic date that evening.

But the next morning, he woke up grumpy and flung my hands away when I tried to touch him; he left me in the bedroom saying he wanted to be alone.

I was very worried and confused; I really thought that something bad had happened to him.

By noon, he was back to his playful, romantic self. I tried to find out what had made him so grumpy earlier but he assured me that everything was fine.

I let it go.

The next day, he threw a tantrum because I sat at his work desk to read a novel. He said his work desk was a 'private and sacred space' and he didn't like anyone going close.

I wondered why he couldn't simply communicate that information to me instead of throwing a tantrum about it.

Saint was like a child, he would get mad and throw tantrums about the stupidest things and hours later, he would be the most amazing boyfriend in the world.

I spent a week in his home but it was exasperating.

I made a decision to play nice until I left and when I get back home, I'll break it off with him. There was no way I was going to be with someone who was so emotionally unstable; just a week together and he was already driving me crazy.

I thought about what the other lady said and I couldn't agree more; he was crazy!!!

I thought it was going to be easy to breakup with him but it wasn't. I was in love with him.

He had a lot of good qualities that were very hard to ignore.

I decided to give the relationship another chance and try harder to make things work- be more patient, ignore his tantrums, and so on.

I felt that if I tried harder, I would be able to change him and get him to be 'normal'

However, as hard as I tried, nothing changed.

I was the one changing- I became angrier, nervous, anxious, and cried every now and then.

I was stuck in an unhealthy relationship.

I called my friend, the bride, who had also known Saint since high school and she confirmed that he had always been a difficult person.

She was the first person to suggest that he probably had some kind of mental health challenge and if I indeed loved him and wanted to be with him, I had to get him help.

I wasn't sure I wanted to stick around with someone who had mental issues but I thought I could at least help him get help before I broke things off with him- that would be my own contribution to his life, I told myself.

I booked an appointment with a mental health professional and I described his character traits and personality to the psychologist.

He told me that I was describing the symptoms of a personality disorder, and that I should encourage them to see a mental health professional for proper diagnosis and treatment. He assured me that it was a treatable condition.

Saint and I have been married for 20 years now and I couldn't have made a better choice. He has been a great husband and the best father to our kids.

After I got him to see a doctor and he started his treatments, he admitted to me that he had dated other women before me and they all left him when they couldn't cope with his mood swings.

People had called him crazy for years but he told me he never felt like he was crazy- he always felt like other people just didn't understand him.

He had a mental health issue and people just tagged him as a person with a bad character- as someone who was just difficult.

No one thought to get him help- they all judged, condemned and abandoned him.

You see, that's the problem with people who suffer from personality disorders- people rarely feel any empathy towards them- they are tagged as difficult people. They are told to get a grip, insulted and avoided.

But would you extend the same treatment to someone who has been diagnosed with cancer?

When a person is diagnosed with cancer, or any other illness, we extend our sympathies to them, we try to help them out, sometimes, we even organize fund raisers to support them.

But when a person has a personality disorder, we treat them with disdain, avoid them and tell them to get a grip.

Personality disorders are just like any other illnesses- something is not right within the patient's body and it is not their fault!

They didn't ask to be born with a personality disorder and they might have no control over the hormonal or chemical imbalances in their brain that is causing them to be so disorganized, moody and imbalanced.

It is not their fault.

And you know the worst thing about the way we treat our friends and family with personality disorders?

They might never get better without the help and support of their family and friends.

Studies have shown that medication alone may not be sufficient enough to manage personality disorders. A combination of family support and medication is more effective than medications alone.

Drugs alone will not help them get better; they need the understanding, help and support of the people around them. They need the people around them to learn how to communicate better with them so that there can be fewer conflicts.

If you had a family or friend who had the flu, would you call them difficult and run away from them?

No, you would make them chicken soup and give them the support and assistance they need to get better.

You won't avoid them or avoid having a relationship with them because they have the flu, or would you?

It's true that people with personality disorders can be very difficult to deal with and frankly, you can lose yourself trying to live or cope with them.

But that's because you don't know how to deal with them just yet.

My relationship with my husband went from toxic and tiring to sweet and loving because I had to learn how to manage his Borderline Personality Disorder.

Today, I'm glad that I didn't throw away all of his good qualities just because he had a disease that he had no control over.

The best way to help your loved one who has been diagnosed with Borderline Personality Disorder is to get familiar with the condition.

Learn about it, and understand what is going on in their head so that you can be fully equipped to manage their condition.

What is Borderline Personality Disorder?

The National Institute of Mental Health defines Borderline Personality disorder as:

"A mental illness that is marked by ongoing patterns of varying moods, self-image, and behaviors that often result in impulsive actions and problems in their relationships."

People with borderline personality disorder will often experience episodes of intense anger, anxiety and depression that can last for a couple of hours or a few days.

People with Borderline Personality Disorder feel like they are on a raft floating on the sea with strong water currents throwing them here and there while they struggle to maintain balance- nothing in their lives feel stable- their moods, behaviors, relationships, thinking, and even their identities are unstable.

Their likes and dislikes will change from time to time and so will their goals.

It's not uncommon for them to have a lot of uncompleted or abandoned projects too because their goals and ambitions can be just as unstable as their moods.

Just like a person with an exposed nerve ending, people suffering from BPD can be so sensitive that those very little things that most people will ignore can trigger intense emotional reactions from them.

There is no middle ground- everything is extreme for them. They feel happy emotions extremely, and unhappy emotions as strongly too.

Another major problem is that when they are upset, they can have a lot of trouble calming down.

They can be very impulsive too- it feels like they take actions now and think about the consequences later.

People who suffer from BPD can also be very clingy and fear abandonment especially because of their previous experiences.

All of these explain why they find it difficult to maintain stable relationships because their emotional instability takes a toll on the people around them, and is easily mistaken for a character flaw.

What Causes Borderline Personality Disorder?

Experts have been unable to pinpoint the exact causes of Borderline Personality Disorder but they have identified a few factors that may be responsible including:

- **Genetics**: Studies have shown that genes inherited from a parent or other family members can increase a person's vulnerability to developing Borderline Personality Disorder.

  One study discovered that there is a 66% chance that if one identical twin has BPD, the other twin will also suffer from the condition.

- **Faulty Brain Development:** Another study conducted on peoples with Borderline Personality Disorder discovered that some parts of their brains were smaller than those of regular people without the disorder.

  Magnetic Resonance Imaging (MRI) scans conducted on their brains revealed that they had smaller:

  - **Hippocampus**: The hippocampus is the part of the brain that helps with self-control and behavior regulation.

○ **Amygdala**: The amygdala is responsible for regulating emotions, especially intense emotions like anxiety, aggression or fear.

○ **Orbitofrontal Cortex:** They also had smaller orbitofrontal cortex, which is the portion of the brain that controls planning and decision making.

The experts believe that these structural defects in the brain may impact the brain's functions, and may be the reason why people with Borderline Personality Disorder have a hard time with all of the functions that these parts of the brain help to coordinate.

• **Chemical Imbalances in the Brain**: In the human brain, there are chemicals known as neurotransmitters. These neurotransmitters help to communicate information from one brain cell to another.

Scientific studies have shown that people with BPD have insufficient neurotransmitters in their brain. Many of them have insufficient serotonin, an important chemical messenger that helps to control destructive urges, aggression or behaviors.

• **Cultural and Social Factors**: A person may develop Borderline Personality Disorder if they've experienced a person who grew up in an unstable home riddled with hostile conflicts may suffer from BPD.

People who have been abused in their childhood or people who suffered abandonment or adversities may develop BPD.

- **Environmental Factors**: Environmental factors may also contribute to development of Borderline Personality Disorder.

  People who grew up in toxic environments can develop BPD. For instance, a person who grew up in a home where an authority figure had a personality disorder or a drug problem can also suffer from BPD.

It doesn't always mean that a person who has been exposed to any of these factors will suffer from the disorder but there are risk factors that can increase a person's chances of suffering from Borderline Personality Disorder.

Symptoms of Borderline Personality Disorder

Some major symptoms of Borderline Personality Disorder include:

- **Inability to Maintain Relationships**: When describing being in a relationship with a BPD patient, a woman said *"One day, everything is fine. Your partner is loving and kind, and the next day, it's awful, and you don't know what hit you. No one really knows what triggered it. It could be because you looked at him or her funny, or you looked at someone else, or you wanted to go somewhere without that person. They perceive abandonment where there is none, and then there is huge rage"*

Prior to my husband, Saint's, diagnosis, dating him was difficult. It was nothing short of a horror story for me, mostly because I often compared my relationship with him with all of my previous relationships.

I had never dated anyone like him and I was convinced that he had a huge problem although I didn't realize it was a medical issue that he had no control over.

I just thought that he was poorly raised, had a secret drug problem or something so I would often yell at him *"Go fix yourself"* as I slam the door in his face or hang up the call during our many arguments.

I really would have dumped him very early into the relationship but the only thing that kept me going was that I saw a side of him that wasn't just sweet but struggling.

I saw that he was struggling to be nicer, to act better but it felt like a force stronger than him was controlling him and forcing him to act badly.

People with Borderline Personality Disorder almost always have difficulties relating with other people. Their romantic relationships are usually short lived even though it's usually intense.

They fall in love quite easily and very fast especially because they see each new love interest as the 'healer'; the one who is going to make them whole but relationships quickly go sour because most people are unable to cope with the emotional rollercoasters that come with dating a BPD patient.

But when you dump them, their fear of abandonment gets worse and the next love interest suffers even more because they believe that person is going to leave too.

o **Terrified of Abandonment:** In the mind of a person suffering from BPD, everyone is going to leave them at some point. It could be due to their previous experiences with abandonment but most patients are often terrified of being left alone.

23

They are usually clingy and will display that fear of abandonment in normal situations like when a partner has to go to work, travel for work, or is late coming back home.

They can start to throw a fit, beg, fight or stalk their loved ones because they fear that the person is trying to leave them.

In the mind of a BPD patient, they are doing all of these because they love you and if anything, they expect you to feel flattered or special but unfortunately; non-patients don't see it that way. Most people just get freaked out by the odd behavior and take to their heels, which further worsen the BPD patient's fear of abandonment.

o **Impulsive Behaviors and Decision-making:** You can't really rely on a BPD patient because even they themselves cannot tell what they can or cannot do.

They often act on impulse, and it's usually like they are being controlled by a force that is greater than them.

One day they are writing budgets and being prudent, the next day they are spending impulsively.

They would also usually engage in other impulsive behaviors like reckless driving, binge-eating, engaging in casual or reckless sex with strangers, abusing alcohol or drugs, or even shoplifting.

Most times, they do these things when they are feeling bad or going through challenges with the hopes that it's going to make them feel better but usually, it just makes them feel even worse.

○ **Shifting Self-image**: BPD patients have no solid sense of self. They can feel great about themselves today- feel like they are smart, intelligent, beautiful, etc. and the next day they think that they suck, they are not good looking, or that they are not doing too well in their careers.

One moment they feel adequate, next minute they want to alter their entire life.

That's why there is a lot of instability in their lives and they will frequently change their jobs, goals, religion, friends, lovers, and sometimes, their sexual orientations.

○ **Engaging in Deliberate Self-harm**: It's not uncommon for patients to have thoughts about harming themselves, or engaging in harmful behaviors like cutting or burning themselves just to inflict pain.

Patients also often have suicidal thoughts and would sometimes threaten to commit suicide or even follow through with it in some cases.

They would also often use suicide as blackmail in relationships when they fear abandonment or rejection.

○ **Short Temper and Explosive Anger**: Another common symptom of Borderline Personality Disorder is short temper that often culminates in explosive anger. Patients are often more impatient than other people and may react with explosive anger to issues that other people might ignore.

o **Emotional Swings and Mood Instability:** This is one of the most common symptoms of Borderline Personality Disorder. A person suffering from this condition would often battle with intense mood swings that they have no control over.

They may feel happy, energetic and anxious (mania) one minute, and the next minute they are feeling despondent, sad, unambitious, lazy, and want to be alone (depression).

o **Feelings of Emptiness:** Patients often describe a feeling of void within them, or feeling empty, and they would usually seek to fill up this void with potentially destructive habits like binge-eating, drug abuse or sex.

o **Intense Paranoia and Feelings of Suspicion:** Paranoia is another common symptom of BPD. They often feel suspicious of other people's intentions and motives, and may start trouble with people or break up friendships for no other reason than suspicion.

They can see a person as good and eulogize the person today, and the next day they're calling the person terrible names and labeling the individual as bad.

○ **Extremist Views and Opinions**: There is often no middle ground for people suffering from BPD. Their views and opinions about issues are often to the extreme, and things would be seen as either of bad or good.

Is Borderline Personality Disorder The Same as Bipolar Disorder?

For effective treatment, it is important to properly diagnose Borderline Personality Disorder; however, a lot of people commonly confuse BPD for Bipolar Disorder.

The conditions are different, and the symptoms and treatments of both conditions are different too.

Bipolar disorder is a mood disorder that causes severe mood swings. People with bipolar disorder will often alternate between depressive mood episodes, and manic mood episodes. They would usually have alternating energy and activity levels, alternating moods, and unstable thoughts.

Mood episodes can last for days or weeks before they change again. During a manic/high energy episode, people suffering from Bipolar disorders will experience:

✓ Sleeping difficulties

✓ Elevated moods

✓ Delusions of grandiose

✓ Grandiose ideas

✓ Exaggerated self-esteem

✓ Optimism towards life and projects in general

✓ Exaggerated self-confidence

✓ Hallucinations

✓ Irritability

✓ Aggression

✓ Recklessness

✓ Impulsive behavior and habits

✓ Racing thoughts and speech

And during a depressive episode they may experience symptoms like:

✓ Fatigue and low energy

✓ Feelings of guilt

✓ Low self-esteem and feelings of worthlessness

✓ Anxiety and excessive worrying

✓ Inability to concentrate

✓ Inability to make decisions

✓ Irritability

- ✓ Withdrawal from society and friends or a desire to be alone

- ✓ Suicidal thoughts

- ✓ Pessimism and indifference

- ✓ Changes in appetite

- ✓ Unexplained tears

- ✓ Loss of interest in hobbies and activities they used to be interested in.

- ✓ Agitation

- ✓ Anger and short temper

- ✓ Changes in sleep patterns

- ✓ Pains and aches

People with BPD suffer from all the symptoms of Bipolar disorder depending on their current moods but they also have problems with their self-image, they have difficulties with interpersonal relationships as well as their thought processes.

Bipolar disorder is mostly a mood disorder although the mood swings can affect other aspects of their lives including their relationships but Borderline Personality Disorder is both a mood disorder and a behavioral or personality disorder.

A personality disorder means that the person struggles with their feelings, thoughts and behaviors and not just their moods.

However, it's possible for a person diagnosed with BPD to also be diagnosed with Bipolar Disorder because dual diagnosis is very common amongst patients.

Dual Diagnosis

Dual diagnosis is when a person suffers from two or more disorders.

Dual diagnosis is very common amongst people living with Borderline Personality Disorder because patients rarely have just BPD disorder. Most patients will often suffer from an accompanying disorder.

Along with BPD, patients can suffer from one of more of the following disorders:

o **Bipolar Disorder**: Extreme mood disorders characterized by alternating episodes of depression and mania.

o **Eating Disorders**: BPD patients often use food as a coping strategy for their alternating moods rather than a source of nourishment, which often leads to eating disorders like Anorexia Nervosa, Binge Eating Disorders or Bulimia Nervosa eating disorder.

o **Addictions**: Patients often have problems with smoking, alcohol and substance abuse too because they also turn to these habits during their depressive episodes and before long, it becomes an addiction that they have no control over.

o **Anxiety Disorders**: BPD patients would often suffer from anxiety attacks or Generalized Anxiety Disorder (GAD).

Everyone gets worried sometimes but BPD patients tend to worry excessively and for trivial things that most people wouldn't even be bothered about. The way they worry about things is also different from other people. Worrying is often intense and characterized by extreme nervousness, anxiety, panic attacks, and tension.

How to Diagnose Borderline Personality Disorder

Getting treatment and healing from Borderline Personality Disorder starts with accepting that there is something wrong with you, and making an appointment with a mental health professional.

But it's hard to find a person suffering from BPD who would agree with you that they have a problem.

As mentioned earlier, BPD is not just a mood disorder but a behavioral disorder. They really don't think that there is anything wrong with the way they are behaving instead; they think that there is something wrong with the other party.

They feel like you are the one who provokes them and makes them act the way they do *"If you didn't say that, I wouldn't have done that"*.

"You know that I don't like when you do this, why did you do it then".

They are never the problem; it's always your fault.

They are often in denial and because of that, they may spend several years battling with this disorder before they are able to get help.

There is also the problem of stigma associated with most mental health disorders. No one wants to be seen as 'sick in the head' or mentally challenged so they would rather continue to struggle than accept that they have a mental health challenge.

Also, the word 'personality disorder' is one that often sounds like there is something wrong with the patient's overall identity and personality so many patients don't take kindly to being tagged as having a personality disorder even though it simply just means that the way that the person relates to the rest of the world is significantly different.

Getting a BPD patient to see that they need to seek help can be a very challenging task but one thing that helps is to get them to answer a simple questionnaire.

The questionnaire can help them see that they have a medical health challenge, and they need help.

		Yes	No
1.	Do you have more than two romantic relationships or friendships that were intense but short-lived?		
	In your relationships, do you often alternate between thinking that a person is wonderful and you love them so much to thinking that they are terrible and you hate them?		
	Do you have intense fears that people will leave or abandon you? Does it often make you act in a way that others might see as a turnoff like stalking them, phoning them excessively, stalking them physically or on social media?		
	Do you engage in self-harm?		

Do you have suicidal thoughts?		
Have you ever tried to commit suicide or have you ever threatened to commit suicide to prevent a person from leaving or breaking up with you?		
Do you ever feel like you don't really know who you are or is your self-image constantly changing?		
Do you engage in any impulsive behavior that can have damaging effects like drug abuse, unsafe sex or impulsive spending?		
Do you have intense mood swings that go from feeling energetic, working hard and feeling very happy to feeling irritable, sad and unwilling to do anything within a couple of hours, days or weeks?		

Do you have feelings of emptiness or loneliness that lasts for a very long time?		
Are you short-tempered and mostly feel like you have no control over your reactions to issues?		
Do you always feel like you overreacted when you cool down after losing your temper?		
Do you have a lot of uncompleted projects that you started when you were feeling happy and energetic but abandoned or lost interest in when your energy levels and mood switched?		

If a person answers 'Yes' to more than 5 of the questions in this questionnaire, the it is an indication that they may be suffering from Borderline Personality Disorder but a visit to a mental health professional will help to put things in clearer perspective.

Borderline Personality Disorder is a Treatable Condition

The good news is that Borderline Personality Disorder is not a life sentence. It is a treatable condition so your friend or loved one doesn't have to live with the condition forever.

We would be discussing some of the effective treatment options for BPD but before we do, let's talk about you.

How do you cope with living with a person living with BPD?

How do you stop them from driving you crazy?

How can you help them get better without losing yourself or your sanity in the process?

That's what we will discuss next.

Chapter 2: How to Help a Person Suffering from Borderline Personality Disorder and Manage Conflicts in the Relationship

To be able to cope with a person suffering from Borderline Personality Disorder, you have to understand their various moods and actions so that you can know what to do to help them at every point in time, and so you can know how to protect yourself and prevent their actions from getting to you.

One of the biggest challenges people with this condition suffer from is mood disorder so it's very important that you learn as much as you can about mood disorders.

What is a Mood Disorder?

We all feel different emotions daily. You can wake up happy and on your way to work something happens that upsets you but by lunch you've already forgotten about it and you're in a good mood again.

Mood fluctuations happen to everyone but when mood fluctuations become so severe that other aspects of your life begins to suffer, especially your work life, relationships, education, and social life, then you may be suffering from a mood disorder

A mood disorder can be defined as *"a serious and constant change in mood that causes disruptions to a person's life activities"*.

Mood disorders are characterized by alternating cycles of elevated mood known as mania or manic episodes and periods of depression. Patients will usually alternate between manic episodes and depressive episodes.

Manic Episodes

A manic episode is when the patient experiences euphoric feelings and high energy. During this phase, they are like Superman-you'd hear them talking about big projects and huge dreams. They are usually very active, happy and creative during this phase.

Although Borderline Personality Disorder patients are pretty much jolly good fellows during a manic episode, their high energy levels can also lead to hyperactivity and impulsiveness. They can indulge in habits that are harmful to them like driving recklessly, spending impulsively, having poor judgment, and overestimating their abilities due to the increased level of optimism they feel during this phase.

If you met your borderline personality disorder lover during a manic episode like I did, you'd easily fall in love with them because they are generally happy and have a positive outlook on life. They would want to go out more, take you to fun places, buy you gifts, do nice things for you and tell you that you're the best thing in the world.

They would hardly pick offence even if someone makes deliberate attempt to hurt them; however, it can come as a rude shock when some days or weeks into the relationship, you begin to see a different side of them that's irritable, quick to anger doesn't want to go out or do anything, is generally moody ad even lazy due to the lower energy levels.

What Causes Mania?

It is difficult to tell what the exact causes of mania are, but experts believe that it is caused by a malfunctioning of the brain chemicals called neurotransmitters.

Neurotransmitters are the chemicals that the brain uses to send messages from one brain cell to another, or from one organ to another.

Neurotransmitters like serotonin, noradrenaline, and dopamine are especially important for regulating moods. They basically tell the brain when to feel pleasure or went to feel unhappy.

Experts believe that patients suffering from borderline personality disorder have malfunctioning neurotransmitters. They liken it to filling your vehicle up with bad gasoline, and even though your vehicle is still running, the bad gasoline is making some parts of the vehicle to malfunction.

Malfunctioning neurotransmitters is believed to be responsible for the severe mood swings. Due to structural or genetic defects in the brain, its ability to regulate neurotransmitters become impacted so at any point in time, the brain chemicals are either too much or too little causing the patient to have intense feelings and energy levels with no middle ground.

People with mood disorders can hardly feel normal; it's either they are extremely happy and active, or extremely sad and too weak to do anything tangible.

What Triggers Manic Episodes?

Manic episodes usually take you by surprise because they often happen without prior warning, and for no particular reason.

However, there are activities that are known triggers of manic episodes. Identifying these triggers can help you prepare for when your loved one might slip into a manic episode.

Some common triggers include:

o Getting too little sleep

o Drinking too much caffeine

o Stress

o Changes in daily routine

o Serious illness

o Loss or death of a loved one

o Alcohol or substance abuse

○ Jet lag from travel

○ Use of antidepressants drugs

Warning Signs of the Onset of a Manic Episode

Because Borderline Personality Disorder patients can sometimes engage in harmful behavior during manic episodes, it is important to look out for them during this period so as to prevent them from doing things that would harm them.

First, you have to learn how to look out for warning signs that they are about to slip into a manic episode.

There a lot of warning signs that can help you tell that they are about to slip into a manic episode so that you can be prepared.

Some of the warning signs include:

○ Suddenly becoming talkative

○ Suddenly expressing ideas that may be deemed unreasonable

○ Sudden short temper or irritability

○ A sudden surge in mood

○ Reckless spending

○ A sudden increase in optimism

How to Take Care of Your Loved One during a Manic Episode

During a manic episode, it's hard to convince your loved one to visit the hospital because this is the time when they often feel good about themselves so it's hard to convince them that feeling good is a problem.

But there are a lot of ways that you can help them manage this high energy period so that it's much more positive for them than negative, and they don't end up harming themselves.

Some of the ways that you can help them:

o Calmly encouraging them to take their medications or visit a healthcare professional.

o Being more observing of their spending habits and discouraging them from making investments or serious financial decisions during this period.

o Encouraging them to journal: journaling can help them keep their thoughts organized, and prevent them from impulsive behaviors.

o Speaking calmly to them especially when they lose their patience. They can be irritable during a manic episode too but don't try to match their irritability with equal anger. Learn how to separate their actions from their personality, and keep in mind that what they are doing at that moment is not their fault but caused by what is happening in their brains that they have no control over.

○ Don't raise your voice when they are raising their voice; instead, speak calmly when they raise their voice – it can help them to also calm down and reason with you. It also helps them to become less irritable.

○ Encourage them to work on their abandoned projects during this phase. As soon as the depressive episode sets in, there is a significant possibility that they would abandon most of the projects that they started to work on during the manic episode so it helps to encourage them to go back to these abandoned projects rather than starting another set of projects.

○ Encourage them to exercise. Exercise goes a long way in helping to regulate the chemicals in the brain and it can be a good way for them to utilize their high energy so that they don't have to engage in potentially dangerous activities.

○ Encourage them to sleep or help them manage their insomnia during this period. Lack of sleep can have severe negative consequences on a person's health so encourage them to get enough sleep. Massage therapy and herbal teas like chamomile are particularly helpful for calming the body down, and inducing sleep.

Depressive Episodes

A depressive episode is the exact opposite of the manic episode. During the depressive phase, the patient feels sad, has low energy, loses interest in things they used to be excited about, and basically withdraws into their shell.

When your loved one switches from a manic episode to a depressive episode, it can seem like you're dealing with two different people living in one body because their attitudes and behaviors are very different.

What Causes Depressive Episodes?

Depressive episodes are also caused by chemical imbalances in the brain or malfunctioning neurotransmitters that make it hard for the brain to regulate moods.

Common Triggers of a Depressive Episode

There are a few things that can trigger depressive episodes even though just like a manic episode, it often happens without warning.

Common triggers include:

o Major life changes especially in their careers or relocation from one place to another.

o Financial difficulties like debts or bankruptcy. Being broke can also trigger a depressive episode in patients.

o Problems in their relationships like rejection, breakups, divorce or a fear of rejection.

o   Loneliness

o   Stress

o   Caffeine

o   Medications

o   Alcohol or drug abuse

Warning Signs of the Onset of a Depressive Phase

There are also a few warning signs that can help you tell that your loved one is about to slip into depression.

Warning signs include:

o   Sudden changes in sleep patterns- they may start to spend longer hours in bed.

o   Sudden withdrawal from society and desire to be alone

o   Sudden loss of interest in hobbies and things they usually enjoy

o   Taking much longer time to complete daily tasks

o   Sluggishness

o   Restlessness and agitation

o   Lack of optimism

o   Changes in appetite and binge-eating

o   Feelings of guilty

o   Sudden increase in irritability

o   Difficulty remembering issues

o   Reduced energy levels

When you begin to notice any of these sudden changes, you can tell that they are about to have a depressive relapse and you can start preparing for it.

How to Care for Your Loved One during a Depressive Phase

It's important to keep an eye on your loved one during this period, even more than the manic episode because thoughts of self-harm and suicide are rife during a depressive phase.

Here are a few helpful ways to care for your loved one during this phase:

o   **Keep Track of Symptoms and Triggers**: It's important to keep a track on what triggers the patient's depressive episodes as spotting the signs early can help to keep their symptoms in check.

o   **Stay Calm**: People with BPD can become difficult to relate with during depressive episodes. They can be slow to anger and irritable so it helps when you stay calm and focus on their strengths rather than their temporary weaknesses.

o **Encourage Breathing Exercises**: Breathing exercises can help to reduce anxiety and reduce the desire for self-harm. Encourage them to take very deep breaths and count from one to ten before exhaling.

Ten reps of breathing exercise at a time can go a long way in helping a person to calm down when they are going through a depressive phase.

o **Plan a Lot of Outdoor Activities**: This is a time when they should be out more and around other people even though they would naturally want to withdraw into their shells and be alone.

You can plan dates, fun activities, and hangouts around this period so that they can be out and around people more, and they can slip out of the depressive phase much faster.

o **Encourage a Healthy Diet**: Depression can trigger the onset of eating disorders because BPD patients often choose food as a coping skill but the brain cells require healthy nutrients to function properly so encourage them to eat a healthy diet so that they have a better chance to snap out of the depressive episode faster.

How to Manage your loved one's Fear of Abandonment

Another important thing you have to learn how to manage when living with or dating a person who suffers from BPD is their fear or abandonment.

Yes, it's mostly baseless- you may not be planning to leave them, and you may not be able to tell why they feel this way but a fear of abandonment is almost always present in the mind of a person who has this disorder.

This fear is sometimes made worse by partners, friends or loved ones who have abandoned them in the past because of the symptoms of their illness.

If you want to help your loved one, you have to know how to manage their fear or abandonment.

o **Ignore Their Outrageous Actions**: BPD patients have a penchant for whipping up trouble when there is none when it comes to issues of abandonment in relationships. They can come up with outrageous accusations like *"Oh, why haven't you been answering your calls, are you trying to leave me?"*

"Why do you have to go on that work trip with a female colleague, are you cheating on me with her?"

And in a bid to try to ensure that you're not leaving them, they can stalk you, get emotional, cry, and try to start fights or eve threaten to commit suicide.

That's just how they are wired- remember that they have a disorder that makes them respond to things differently than other regular people. So, you would have to learn how to ignore the outrageous things that they do, and recognize it as a temporary symptom of an illness because as soon as they start getting treatment and therapy, they would become better at managing their fears of abandonment.

○ **Reassure Them Constantly**: When they express their fear of abandonment, whether directly or indirectly through negative behavior, what you should do is to reassure them.

Look beyond the negative behavior.

Like when they start accusing you of cheating or trying to dump them, just take a deep breath to calm yourself, hold their hands and look into their eyes, then offer some sweet words of reassurance like *"I know you think I'm going to leave you like the others, but trust me, I'm here for the long haul. Even though things are not perfect in our relationship right now, I'm ready to make it work because I love you. Please, always trust me even when you don't understand my actions, I love you and I will never do anything to hurt you"*.

You can say it to them or you can send it in a text or a mail- it will go a long way in allaying their fears or abandonment, and in helping them feel more relaxed about the relationship and this ultimately leads to fewer conflicts in the relationship.

o **Don't Play Mind Games**: Most people play mind games in relationships to try to gain the upper hand but if you're with someone who has the Borderline Personality Disorder, you have to keep it straight and real in the relationship because they don't have the bandwidth to handle emotional rollercoasters or uncertainty in relationships.

Don't try to withdraw from them to make them miss you, or ignore their calls, or flaunt someone else just to make them jealous- people with BPD usually have a problem with handling mind games so just keep it straight and real with them.

o **Always Keep in Touch**: Don't leave your BPD lover or friend for days without getting in touch. Because of their fear of abandonment, they have the need to stay connected to the people they love.

How to Manage Conflicts in the Relationship

Conflict management is another important aspect you have to pay attention to when you have a loved one who suffers from Borderline Personality Disorder.

Finger pointing and blame games would not help, what can help you get along and live peacefully with a person who suffers from this condition is learning how to relate with one another in a healthy way.

I'll share a few tips that helped me manage the constant conflicts my partner and I had, and how we were able to restore the peace and sanity in our relationship.

○ **Don't Feed The Drama:** It takes two to fight and argue. Yes, BPD patients are a pain in the neck, and they are just impossible but have you ever seen a person fighting with themselves?

For a conflict to really happen, it has to take the involvement of both parties.

It can feel unfair, like why do you have to be the bigger one but, you already know that this person has a medical challenge that is the reason why they are behaving that way so engaging with them is like pouring fire into a volcano; it doesn't help.

One tool that personally employed is humor- when my husband starts throw tantrums, I already anticipate it and I just make a joke and then we both end up laughing about it.

It will help to reduce the conflicts in your relationships if you can avoid engaging them or matching their actions when they try to start fights with you.

○ **Don't Make Promises You Cannot Keep:** We already talked about this- BPD sufferers are not too good at handling uncertainties and disappointments so it's best to avoid making promises that you can't keep to them and in circumstances where disappointments are unavoidable, take your time to explain to them. Being nonchalant about disappointments can trigger anger feats and tantrum episodes.

- o **Set Boundaries and Establish Rules**: You don't have to take everything that they throw at you; it's okay to establish rules and boundaries.

When they start 'going too far' or engaging in behaviors that are potentially harmful to you or those that are unacceptable, it's okay to calmly inform them that their behavior is unacceptable.

- o **Take Time to Disengage**: Giving each other space is also a very helpful way to deescalate conflicts. It's okay to walk away or take some time off if you feel overwhelmed.

Don't threaten to abandon them; you calmly tell them their actions are affecting you right now, and you think that both of you need some space from each other at the moment.

If you're taking time off, make sure you reassure them that you are not abandoning them but simply taking a break to help both of you cool off so you don't trigger their fears of abandonment.

- o **Don't Force Them to Talk**: After a conflict, normal people would want to talk about it, and maybe kiss and make up but for a person with BPD, they may not feel like talking immediately and forcing them to talk might just trigger another set of conflicts.

It is important to allow them to calm down and process their thoughts and feelings properly before talking about issues; otherwise, nothing they say at that moment is going to help- they'll only just make things worse.

- o **Be Empathetic**: Showing empathy can help to reduce conflicts or prevent them before they even start.

Saying kind and soothing words like *"I know how you feel, I'm sorry you feel this way"* before asserting your opinions or stands on issues can go a long way.

Chapter 3: Effective Treatments and Therapies for Borderline Personality Disorder

Borderline Personality disorder can be a scary condition- no one wants to be stuck with someone who is so unstable for the rest of their lives.

But you don't have to because it is not a permanent condition. Many people stick with the condition for longer than usual only because they couldn't identify that there is a problem and get a diagnosis early enough.

Once your loved one has been diagnosed, there are a lot of therapies and treatments that can help them improve and start to get better immediately.

Some of the effective treatments and therapies for Borderline Personality Disorder include:

Psychotherapy

Psychotherapy for Borderline Personality Disorder is also known as Talk Therapy. It involves the use of interpersonal or group interaction to try to change a person's behaviors and teach them better ways to interact with other people and handle the challenges they face with their moods, self-image, and thought process.

There are a lot of psychotherapy methods that are used to treat Borderline Personality Disorder but the most effective ones include:

✓ **Dialectal Behavior Therapy**

Dialectal Behavior Therapy also known as DBT, is a psychotherapy that helps to teach the patient healthy ways to cope with stress, manage conflicts, regulate their emotions, and improve their relationships.

It can also help to prevent destructive behaviors and eating disorders in people suffering from BPD.

Dialectal Behavior therapy was first introduced in the late 80's by Dr. Mashan Linehan, after discovering that Cognitive Behavioral Therapy(CBT), which commonly worked for people suffering from other personality disorders, was not effective for people suffering from Borderline Personality Disorder.

Dialectal Behavior Therapy is based on the concept of Dialectics, which is a belief that for every force, there is an opposing force that is stronger.

Patients are made to understand that:

- ○ Change is inevitable and constant

- ○ Everything is connected

- ○ Opposing forces can come together to bring out positive results

People who suffer from BPD often have problems dealing with changes and opposing ideas, actions or personalities so this therapy teaches them how to embrace and manage changes, and help them to see that change is inevitable and an inherent quality of life itself.

Patients are also taught how to validate other people's opinions and ideas without necessarily accepting that it is the best approach.

Rather than throw tantrums because you said that Pizza is a better dinner than burger, they would be able to 'respect' your opposing ideas and opinions without necessarily accepting or adopting it.

Dialectal Behavior therapy is one of the most effective treatments for Borderline Personality Disorder and it is often done through group sessions, phone coaching and one on one therapy.

✓ Schema-Focused Therapy (SCT)

Schema-focused therapy helps patients to identify negative behaviors and patterns that they might have developed over time as a coping skill for Borderline Personality Disorder.

For instance, an adult who has suffered from BPD from when they were a child could have developed some negative traits like maybe binge-eating or snapping at people or being too clingy in order to prevent people from abandoning them.

Schema-focused therapy helps to identify these negative coping skills, and helps the patient to learn new, positive coping skills.

✓ Mentalization-based Therapy (MBT)

Another therapy that teaches BPD patients positive coping skills is Mentalization-based Therapy.

Patients are taught how to chart their own thoughts and feelings, and identify what they may be feeling at any point in time so that they can properly ponder on issues before reacting.

BPD patients are prone to impulsive habits and actions- they often react before they think unlike the rest of us who would often think about our actions and reactions carefully before letting them out.

Mentalization-based therapy basically helps patients to think and reflect on the consequences of their actions before acting them out.

✓ Transference-focused Psychotherapy (TFP)

Transference-focused psychotherapy is really great for BPD patients who are married or in romantic relationship, and want to improve their relationship with their partner.

The psychotherapist teaches the patient how to understand their emotions and develop good interpersonal relationship that the patient can duplicate with other people.

All of these therapies are effective and patients can choose one or a combination of therapies depending on what their problem areas are.

However, you would need the help of a mental healthcare professional or a psychologist to recommend the best therapy for the individual.

o **Medications**: Drugs like antidepressants, mood stabilizers, and antipsychotics are very helpful too especially for reducing symptoms like depression, anxiety, aggressiveness, and impulsiveness.

A doctor can prescribe medications to be used along with therapy because medications alone may only have temporary effects while a combination of both can provide permanent relief from Borderline Personality Disorder.

o **Hospitalization**: Hospitalization may be necessary where the patient may be suicidal or engaging in self-harm. They would have to be hospitalized and placed on suicide watch where they can start to take medications and therapies that would help to improve their condition.

o **Self-help**: There are a lot of ways that a person suffering from Borderline Personality Disorder can help themselves outside medications and therapies.

Some helpful self-help strategies include:

▪ **Breathing Exercises**: Breathing exercises help you calm down by sending signals to your sympathetic nervous system that is responsible for coordinating your flight or fight response.

Learning how to breathe, especially during distressful situations can help to prevent interpersonal conflicts.

Instead of responding impulsively, the patient can cultivate a habit of taking quick, deep breaths before responding to any situation.

It will not only help them calm down, but also help them ponder on actions before acting them out.

- **Journaling and Mood-charting**: The brain of a person with Borderline Personality Disorder can be likened to that of a little child. A little child is yet to understand why they are feeling a certain way, and they can't express their feelings so they would cry, throw tantrums and lash out all the time.

But if the child is able to identify what he or she is feeling at that moment, they can easily say "I'm hungry' rather than cry until you ask them if they want food.

Mood-charting can help a patient anticipate and identify their feelings at any point in time, so that they can avoid 'punishing' other people instead of looking inwards and tackling the issue from within them.

Mood-charting can be done with a pocket notebook, where the patient would have to record their moods and feelings at every hour of the day for a period of time, maybe a couple of weeks or months.

After some time, a pattern would emerge and it will be easy to tell how and what the patient may feel at different periods.

The patient would also be able to prepare themselves to handle the people and challenges that they are likely to come across during these periods.

o **Family Therapy**

The truth is that it is the family and friends that suffer most. If you are living with someone who suffers from BPD, it can take a negative toll on you and since the condition can be passed on to people who grew up or lived with BPD patients for a long time, your children may be at risk of developing Borderline Personality disorder too.

Family therapy is not only helpful for learning how to cope with, and live with patients without conflicts, it can also be a preventive or protective measure for people who have to live with or relate with a person who has the Borderline Personality Disorder.

Family therapy involves all members of the household working together with a therapist. You would all attend sessions as a group, where you would be taught how to communicate and cope with the patient, and how to avoid dangerous BPD family cycles from forming.

You would also be taught how to set boundaries and take care of yourself while caring for your loved one.

Family therapy is often more effective than individual therapy because the patient will still face difficulties at home if family and friends don't know how to communicate and live with them until their condition improves.

There are a lot of family therapy programs for Borderline Personality Disorder but a very common and effective one is Systems Training for Emotional Predictability and Problem-solving (STEPPS). It is a 20-week program that all family members have to attend. The program helps you learn how to predict the patient's reactions to common issues, and help you learn positive ways to respond, communicate and live with them.

Recovery Takes Time

Your loved one will get better as soon as they start receiving treatments but it is important to note that this will not happen overnight.

Some patients will get better almost immediately, while some might take years to respond to recovery so make sure you are patient with your loved one, and you give them as much time as they need to get better.

Chapter 4: How to Take Care of Yourself and Avoid Losing Your Sanity While Dealing with a Person with Borderline Personality Disorder

All along, we've been talking about how to take care of your partner who has Borderline Personality Disorder but what about you?

Borderline Personality Disorder definitely takes its toll on the partner and family members. In fact, you are the ones who bear the brunt in the relationship because you have to be the bigger one all the time.

You have to ignore a lot of things and be emotionally strong because a lot of what your partner does can hurt you and drive you crazy.

So how do you take care of yourself to ensure that you don't lose it while living with, and loving a person who has Borderline Personality Disorder?

Understand Some of the Ways That Their Illness Can Affect You, and Be Prepared for Them

The first key to caring for yourself is anticipating the difficulties. It's easier to deal with the issues when you already expect or know what would happen.

Living with a person who has Borderline Personality Disorder can affect the partner and the family in a number of ways including:

1. Disruption in Regular Routines

Their mood is hardly stable and so are their desires. You could have planned to attend a family event together during the weekend and when the day comes, your partner decides that they want to stay back at home to watch soccer, or they would rather spend the day with a friend instead.

All of this is bound to get to you, and make you really angry because, how do you tell your mom and dad that he's no longer coming? And for what? Because he wants to hang out with a random stranger instead?

The truth is that, when dealing with someone who has the borderline personality disorder, you have to be flexible, both in your expectations of them, and in what you tell others that they would do.

Even when your partner has promised and swears that they would do something, always have it at the back of your mind that it's possible that they won't be able to do it, not because they don't want to, but because they have a temporary illness that prevents them from taking full control of their actions and decisions.

2. Financial Difficulties

Impulsive behaviors are common with people who suffer from this disorder and impulsive spending is one of the most challenging of their impulsive tendencies.

Your partner can make a mess of the family's finances if they are given total control. You may soon find yourself dealing with a lot of debt repayments due to financial recklessness on your partner's part.

Whilst it may be difficult for you to ask your partner not to do whatever they like with their own money, you can encourage them to use a budget to plan expenditure.

A budget can go a long way in preventing impulsive spending.

3. Changes in Traditional Family Roles

Another problem you may experience in the relationship is the frequent changes in family roles.

Traditionally, the man is like the head or the authority figure in the home- he protects his family, makes decisions and basically, takes charge of the home. The woman on the other hand, is the one who cooks the meals, tends to the household, and takes care of the kids, and so on.

Not trying to be misogynistic here but these are the traditional roles in most households.

But when dealing with a person who has the disorder, you can find yourself switching roles, and standing in for them a lot of times.

She may wake up one morning and decide that she doesn't want to get out of bed that day while she is supposed to be the one who preps the kids for school. So, you would have to step in and fulfill her responsibilities for that day.

A child who has a parent that has Borderline Personality Disorder might find themselves being the caretaker and decision maker a lot of times whereas, it's usually the other way round.

You have to be prepared for these traditional role reversals so as to keep the family functioning; otherwise, the family may become dysfunctional.

4. Health Problems Due to Stress

Until you learn how to deal with, and relate with your BPD partner in a healthy way, the emotional stress is inevitable.

The problem however, is that emotional stress can lead to other physical symptoms like elevated blood pressure, headaches, sleeping difficulties, and headaches amongst others.

Research has also shown that emotional stress can make already existing illnesses become even worse.

The emotional stress that family members experience when living with a person who has Borderline Personality Disorder can trigger other health problems that may cost a lot of money and time to treat.

5. Dangerous or Reckless Behavior

A friend whose husband also has Borderline Personality Disorder shared her experience with me about how her husband came home drunk one day while she was at work, took the kids from the nanny, put them in the car, and took them on a long reckless drive on the highway.

They got into an accident and even though the kids were unhurt, the man had to go to jail for reckless endangerment.

This is a perfect example of how dangerous behavior triggered by Borderline Personality Disorder can put not just the patient's life, but every other family member's life at risk.

We've heard gory stories of BPD partner's starting fires, flinging babies, and putting their family members through all sorts of risks in a fit of rage.

Don't Encourage Co-dependency

You don't have to put your life on hold because your partner suffers from this illness.

Set boundaries in your relationship and be strict with it.

The relationship shouldn't become so unhealthy that their actions begin to infringe on your life, your goals, and your wellbeing.

You have every right to happiness, career fulfillment, dreams, ambitions and everything you have planned out for yourself, even if you are in a relationship with someone who suffers from Borderline Personality Disorders.

So, don't put your life on hold for them. There's nothing wrong with making yourself a priority.

Although they have an illness, people with Borderline Personality Disorder are not incapable of making conscious decisions to improve upon their habits and actions especially when it's one that affects you negatively.

If they are not willing to make efforts to look out for you, then it's hard for you to continue to be the only one looking out for your partner.

If their illness begins to affect your life negatively, consider going for some relationship counseling, where you can 'nicely' make them become aware of how their actions are affecting you and how they might leave you no choice but to leave.

Don't Ignore Threats

It's true that people with this disease make a lot of empty threats, mostly to get attention or blackmail you emotionally but the problem is that, you can never tell when they are bluffing or when they are indeed serious.

This is why you can't afford to ignore any threats. If they start threatening, talk to them calmly, and if they don't calm down, dial 911 or any emergency service number in your locality.

Walk Away From Harmful Behavior

Some patients may have violent tendencies and may harm you during an argument.

First, it's important to avoid arguments with them but if they are still violent, the first thing you should do is to take cover.

It's important to protect yourself first because you're dealing with someone who is mentally unwell.

Take cover and call the police in if they start throwing things, wielding a knife, or behaving in a way that may put other people at risk.

Let the Children Understand What is Going On

Kids shouldn't begin to take their Borderline Personality Disorder parent's actions and behaviors as the norm.

If there are children in the house, you have to make them understand that *"Daddy/mommy is not acting normally because Daddy/mommy has a sickness"*.

Since BPD traits can be passed on to children, it's best to be proactive with your kid's response to the situation.

This is not something you hide from them; be open with them about the illness, and make sure they attend family therapy sessions too.

Take Frequent Breaks from Your Partner

Until your partner gets better, or at least until you master the skills of communicating and living in peace with a person who has Borderline Personality Disorder, you're going to be going through a lot of emotional stress, which can quickly translate to physical stress.

It therefore becomes important for you to take time off regularly to de-stress.

This is called loving detachment.

You can go for spa trips, visit friends or family, go on solo-trips or dates- just make sure you spend some time away from them as often as you can where you can get some massage, some long walks, and other things that can help you rejuvenate.

Go for Personal Therapy Sessions and Counseling

It's not just your partner that needs therapy, you do too. You may not realize it but dealing with a BPD patient can impact your mental health negatively too.

It helps to have a therapist that you can vent to, talk about your challenges with, and basically help you with any emotional or mental tension that may build up as you deal with your partner.

Trust me, it helps to keep you calm, and goes a long way in keeping you from going crazy.

Encourage Responsibility

Don't indulge them every time they do something bad; it's not helpful when you do that.

If they break something during a fit of rage, don't replace it.

If every time you visit, it ends up with fights and arguments, don't visit anymore and let them know that though you love them, it's difficult for you to be around them when all you do is fight.

This way, you're encouraging them to be responsible and focus more on getting better.

This way, you would also be protecting your own happiness and sanity.

Don't Give in to Manipulation

People who suffer from Borderline Personality Disorder are often master manipulators.

With them, you can easily find yourself saying yes to a lot of things that you would have preferred to say no to.

This might leave you feeling unhappy with yourself, or having to put yourself through a lot of discomfort just to give them what they want.

You can't live that way because it's not healthy for you- it's okay to establish rules and go with what's comfortable for you.

You don't have to be mean or rude about it; just explain to them as nicely as you can.

Say something like *"I understand how you feel, I know you've not had steak in a while but we can't afford that right now because the rent is due tomorrow. I'm sure that by next week, we would be able to afford all the steaks we want".*

Be assertive but in a kind and considerate way.

Conclusion

"No good deed goes unpunished".

That's how it feels when dealing with someone who has Borderline Personality Disorder.

It's like you can never win with them, no matter what you do.

But remember, it's not their fault.

They didn't choose to be born with a brain defect that makes it difficult for them to regulate their thoughts, emotions and actions.

However, this is not something that they have to live with forever.

Yes, there are people who live with this disorder throughout their lifetimes but most people who do, are unaware that they have a personality disorder.

These days, there are a lot of effective treatment plans for patients that can put the illness in check.

The best thing you can do for your spouse/partner/friend/coworker who suffers from this condition is to help them seek treatment. You also have to understand the illness, learn how to communicate with them and de-escalate conflicts, and learn how to protect yourself both physically and mentally while dealing with them.

With all of these, your relationship with your partner will go from toxic and problematic, to peaceful and happy.

Do You Like My Book & Approach To Publishing?

If you like my writing and style and would love the ease of learning literally everything you can get your hands on from Fantonpublishers.com, I'd really need you to do me either of the following favors.

1: First, I'd Love It If You Leave a Review of This Book on Amazon.

2: Check Out Some Books On Emotional Mastery

Emotional Intelligence: The Mindfulness Guide To Mastering Your Emotions, Getting Ahead And Improving Your Life

Stress: The Psychology of Managing Pressure: Practical Strategies to turn Pressure into Positive Energy (5 Key Stress Techniques for Stress, Anxiety, and Depression Relief)

Failure Is Not The END: It Is An Emotional Gym: Complete Workout Plan On How To Build Your Emotional Muscle And Burning Down Anxiety To Become Emotionally Stronger, More Confident and Less Reactive

Subconscious Mind: Tame, Reprogram & Control Your Subconscious Mind To Transform Your Life

Body Language: Master Body Language: A Practical Guide to Understanding Nonverbal Communication and Improving Your Relationships

Shame and Guilt: Overcoming Shame and Guilt: Step By Step Guide On How to Overcome Shame and Guilt for Good

Anger Management: A Simple Guide on How to Deal with Anger

Get updates when I publish any book that will help you master your emotions: http://bit.ly/2fantonpubpersonaldevl

To get a list of all my other books, please check out my author profile or let me send you the list by requesting them below: http://bit.ly/2fantonpubnewbooks

3: Grab Some Freebies On Your Way Out; Giving Is Receiving, Right?

I gave you a complimentary book at the start of the book. If you are still interested, grab it here.

5 Pillar Life Transformation Checklist: http://bit.ly/2fantonfreebie

Made in the USA
Coppell, TX
26 August 2021